Ultimate Coconut Oil Guide!

Coconut Oil

Coconut Oil Recipes For Organic Skin Care And Natural Beauty, Clean Eating For Weight Loss, Shinning Hair, Better Brain Function And Overall Health!

Sarah Brooks

STOP!!! Before you read any further….Would you like to know the secrets of Anti-Aging?

If your answer is yes, then you are not alone. Thousands of people are looking for the secret to reducing wrinkles, looking younger, and maintaining a youthful appearance.

If you have been searching for these answers without much luck, you are in the right place!

Not only will you gain incredible insight in this book, but because I want to make sure to give you as much value as possible, right now for a limited time you can get full **100% FREE access to a VIP bonus EBook** entitled **Anti-Aging Made Easy!**

Just Go Here For Free Instant Access:

www.LuxyLifeNaturals.com

Legal Notice

Disclaimer Notice

Table Of Contents

Introduction

I want to thank you and congratulate you for purchasing the book, *Coconut Oil: Ultimate Coconut Oil Guide! - Coconut Oil Recipes for Organic Skin Care and Natural Beauty, Clean Eating for Weight Loss, Shining Hair, Better Brain Function and Overall Health!*

This book contains proven steps and strategies on how you can take full advantage of the beauty, weight loss and health benefits that coconut oil has to offer. Through this book, you will learn more about:

1. What makes coconut oil healthy?
2. How it can help you get better, more glowing skin.
3. Its effects on your hair and making healthier.
4. Can coconut oil improve your brain function?
5. Weight loss benefits and how it can boost your metabolism.
6. Coconut oil and how it can help treat different illnesses.
7. Recipes for both your diet as well as organic skin care.
8. How to choose the right coconut oil for your needs.

We hope that through this book, you'll be able to recognize the amount of potential that a single bottle of coconut oil contains.

Thanks again for purchasing this book, I hope you enjoy it!

Chapter 1: Coconut Oil For Natural Beauty And Health

These days, more and more people are becoming aware of the effects that chemically manufactured products has on their bodies. As such, many of them have turned to a greener, more organic lifestyle that advocates going all natural when it comes to their food as well as the different products that they use on their bodies.

This isn't surprising, of course, considering the fact that there are a number of illnesses which are associated with constant use of synthetic and often chemical-laden skin and health products. There are certain risks that one must bear when using it; risks which can be avoided altogether if one were to switch over to something that's a bit closer to nature.

The coconut oil is a favorite among health buffs as it is one of those by-products that can be used in a multitude of ways. On one hand, it can be eaten and taken as a supplement which would boost your overall health. On the other, it can be applied topically and used as a beauty product as well as a means of treating certain skin issues.

You get all of these benefits but without worrying about its harmful effects to the body.

Why is it considered one of the best natural remedies out there?

It's all in the composition. About 99% of it is composed of saturated fats (which, in this case isn't as bad as it sounds) as well as traces of polyunsaturated fatty acids and mono saturated fatty acids. Virgin coconut oil retains a higher amount of the good stuff thus it is also valued higher.

It also contains lauric acid and quite a generous amount of it at that. When digested by the body, this would turn into mono laurin and is very beneficial when it comes to dealing with different bacteria and viruses. Diseases such as influenza and herpes are just two of the things that coconut oil can cure in a jiff. A tablespoon of it a day keeps the doctor away, so to speak.

Besides these, it is also one of the most powerful inhibitors of quite a number of different pathogenic organisms ranging from your usual viruses to even protozoa. All of this, of course, is attributed to its high lauric acid content.

For beauty and skincare

Coconut can also be used for cosmetic or skin care purposes. We'll get to the specifics of this in later chapters but to quickly summarize, it is often used for: Hair care, skin care, nails, lips as well as treating different skin issues such as psoriasis. It helps keep the skin youthful and glowing as well as protect it from harmful UV rays.

Chapter 2: Coconut Oil For Healthy And Shining Hair

When it comes to beauty products, many would tell you that natural options remain the best when it comes to long-term effects. They are known to be less harsh on your hair and at the same time, nourish it with constant use. However, there are very few products out there that can be considered a cure-all. For that, all you need to do is grab a bottle of coconut oil for yourself. Trust us when we say, most of what you need is already in it.

Hollywood celebrities swear by it when it comes to keeping their hair beautiful and healthy. Here's how you can have some of that for yourself.

Coconut oil is one of the most inexpensive treatments for your hair currently available and the best bit? It is all natural. In fact, many people say that it is much better than other treatments in the market. Those that contain alcohol and silicone do tend to damage the hair and its roots with continuous use. Some experience skin allergies from using it too much. Needless to say, there are certain risks that one must consider, but with coconut oil, there isn't any.

Here are some of the ways you can use coconut oil for your hair:

As a deep conditioner – If your hair is over-processed, damaged, frizzy and extremely brittle due to dryness, then it's about time you took matters in your own hands. For a fraction of what it would cost to get salon treatments, you can bring back vitality into your hair just by massaging a tablespoon of coconut oil into it at least twice a week. You will need more of it if you have thicker or longer hair and with some experimentation, you should be able to find the right amount for yourself.

As a detangler/moisturizer – If your hair is a little on the curly side, you would know how tangled the ends can become after you shower. Instead of damaging your hair further with a detangling comb which forces your hair apart, just smooth in some coconut oil into it after you shower. Work it thoroughly into the ends before gently and slowly combing out the knots.

For dandruff treatment – Anti dandruff shampoos can leave your hair feeling dry sometimes and they don't really work on the cause of the problem which is a dry scalp. Most of the time, these shampoos only get rid of visible flakes and nothing more. Instead, opt for some coconut oil. Massage it onto your scalp this time and allow to sit for half an hour or even overnight. Just make sure that you wear a shower cap to make sure it doesn't get on your pillows. Do it twice a week and you'll soon see a big difference.

Chapter 3: Coconut Oil For Organic Skin Care

Coconut oil contains certain components which are beneficial to our skin as well. For example, it contains vitamin E which is known to help in skin growth, skin repair, moisturizing, nourishing and best of all, it also helps in preventing premature skin aging. The proteins in it are also great for your skin, keeping it rejuvenated from the inside to the outside. Besides that, it also contributes to continuous cell and tissue repair which helps make sure that your skin remains youthful looking and any signs of sagging can be remedied. Here are some of the ways you can use it for your skin:

As a moisturizer – Coconut oil is one of the best natural moisturizers available out there. It will keep your skin properly nourished as well as keep it from drying up quickly. All you need is a few drops of it then work it into your skin. Many spas also use this particular oil for aromatherapy massages given the fact that it has a relaxing and warming effect on the skin which your average lotion cannot provide you with. Use it on your body and even your face without worry.

As a lip balm – If you look up what comprises a natural lip balm, it wouldn't be surprising if you spot coconut oil as one of its ingredients. Coconut oil is a great remedy for cracked and chapped lips. After all, you can't just use any old product on it considering the fact that there is a great chance that you might swallow it when you lick your lips. Remember, there are preservatives and chemicals in non-natural lip treatments so you might want to think twice about using them.

As an exfoliant – Typical exfoliates can leave your skin feeling raw and damaged. At times, it can also block your pores thus causing more irritation and problems. This isn't the case if you use coconut oil. If used in conjunction with gentle exfoliates such as sugar, it will be a soothing experience and would leave your skin glowing and even colored. You don't even need to worry about getting your pores clogged because as you exfoliate, everything gets dissolved and absorbed into your skin thus nourishing it even more.

As a treatment for skin disorders – Problems such as eczema, acne and psoriasis can be easily treated with the use of coconut oil. Of course, depending on the extent, it might take longer for some people to see changes. What coconut oil does is heal and repair the broken skin. It hastens the process of replacing the dead and damaged skin cells with newer, healthier ones. Any visible marks such as acne scars can also diminish in time with constant use of coconut oil. Even the act of massaging it onto your skin helps; it brings oxygenated blood into the area, helping with the process of healing even more.

When it comes to beauty and taking care of your skin, a single bottle of coconut oil will certainly go a long way. In this respect, you're actually staying healthy and saving money at the same time.

Chapter 4: Fat Loss, Faster Metabolism And Clean Eating

Can coconut oil really help you lose weight? The answer would be, yes. It can help you lose weight through its own unique combination of different fatty acids, all of which have powerful effects on the metabolism. In fact, a number of studies have been done on this subject and many of them all concluded that coconut oil can help you get rid of excess fat, especially the ones in the abdominal cavity-- often deemed to be dangerous to your health.

But how exactly does it work? Allow us to show you three different ways through which coconut oil can help you lose weight.

Boosts your metabolism. While it may contain fat, these are vastly different from the ones you may typically find in other foods. On average, the food that you consume is predominantly comprised of LCFA's or long chain fatty acids. These take much longer to break down and are also one of the most common causes of dietary issues. Coconut oil, on the other hand, consists of MCFA's or medium chain fatty acids which are easily metabolized by the body and turned into energy.

MCFA's are sent straight to your liver where they would then be converted into ketone bodies or as energy to help power you throughout the day. This allows your body to work at quicker pace thus boosting your metabolism. The faster your metabolic rate is, the more fats you burn.

Now, let's talk calories. You have to keep in mind that not all calories are the exact same. Different foods as well as macronutrients would go through a number of metabolic pathways and the outcomes are never the same. Some metabolic pathways tend to be more efficient than others which there are those that take more energy just so you can digest and then metabolize them. This is also why you should be mindful of what you eat. Steaks, for one, fall under the slow metabolizing category. As such, you may want to eat less of it.

It has thermogenic properties. This particular property of the coconut oil sets it apart from other types of fats. What this does is increase the fat burning or energy expenditure that your body does. In simpler terms, it boosts your metabolism, thus making your body more efficient at burning fats from food items such as steaks. One study showed that for about 2 tablespoons of coconut oil, you can increase your energy expenditure by at least 5% which totals to about 120 calories each day. That's quite a lot, isn't it? Considering you didn't do much work besides consume some coconut oil.

So are calories from coconut oil the same as the ones found in olive oil? Not by a long shot. They are not the same kind of calories but, you'll be glad to know that both are good for your overall health.

Helps reduce your appetite. Studies have shown that medium fatty acids can help increase feelings of being full after eating. Of course, this would then help you avoid overeating which leads to a reduction in your calorie intake. This can also be related to the way the fats are being metabolized. It is a known fact that ketone bodies (produced by your liver when you consume coconut oil) do have a significant appetite-reducing effect.

So there you have it, a three step process through which coconut oil can help you lose weight and eat healthier. You don't have to consume a huge amount of it because much like other good stuff, it still needs to be taken in moderation.

Chapter 5: Coconut Oil For Better Brain Function

Can coconut oil actually improve brain function? Studies have shown that, yes, it certainly is capable of it. To understand how it works, however, we have to start from the beginning.

Currently, there are about 5.4 million people in America who have Alzheimer's disease. This is a type of dementia that brings about thinking, memory and behavioral problems. The symptoms typically develop slowly, gradually growing worse over time to the point where it becomes a hindrance to a person's everyday life. It is, for many, a scary thought to even imagine happening to themselves.

There are very few treatments for it and they are rarely effective. This is one of the reasons as to why doctors always put emphasis on early diagnosis as well as prevention. For that, coconut oil just might be one of the best defenses that we have. What studies have put forth is the idea that this particular oil is the ideal brain food for people – alternative fuel for your brain which is also much healthier than the usual; it is even healthy enough to help prevent the onset of Alzheimer's.

But how does it work?

There are two different fuel types that the body is capable of converting into energy. These would be: carbs/sugar or fat. Ketones, on the other hand, are produced when the body converts fat into energy. As we have previously tackled, MCT's are the primary source of ketones for the body and what's the best natural source for it? Coconut oil. So what has that got to do with Alzheimer's and better brain function?

While the brain is perfectly content with using glucose as fuel, there are evidence which suggests that we can further improve it as well as keep it healthy. Ketone bodies, as studies have shown, are capable of renewing and restoring neurons as well as proper nerve function in the brain even after some damage has begun. The interesting thing here is that this entire process of MCT-ketone metabolism happens because your body begins treating MCT's as a carbohydrate as opposed to being a fat.

But the best bit about the MCT-ketone metabolism process is that it allows the ketone energy to enter your bloodstream without affecting your insulin levels. In effect, coconut oil acts as a carb when it comes to fuelling your brain. A much healthier alternative to the usual, don't you think?

Chapter 6: Coconut Oil And The Right Brain Diet

So what kind of diet is needed when it comes to keeping your brain healthy and functioning efficiently? Other than coconut oil, you also need to make sure that your diet is rich in different ingredients that sustain ketones. Here are some of the supplements you might want to include in your everyday diet:

Coconut Oil – Just how much of it do you need? Studies show that 20 grams of MCT a day should be more than enough fuel for your brain and for that, you will need 2 tablespoons of coconut oil daily. You can add it to your favorite dishes, to your coffee, breakfast oats or take it straight up, without additives. It depends on your preference and taste, of course. The best variety would be the virgin coconut oil and though a bit pricier than the usual, it also retains more of the good stuff.

Glucose – Glucose is the brain's primary source of energy and of course, without it, it will eventually undergo a cognitive decline. Soon, the person will experience problems with their memory as well as thinking. Ketones are an alternative energy source but these two can also work in conjunction with each other. Of course, balance is important in this case.

Other "Brain foods" to add to your regular diet:

Wild salmon (and other deep-water fish) – These are rich in omega-3 essential fatty acids which play a vital role when it comes to proper brain function. Wild salmon is recommended by experts due to its cleanliness as well as the fact that it is plentiful. Sardines and herring are two other varieties of fish that you may want to start eating more of. A 4-ounce serving, eaten 2 to 3 times a week should provide you with what your brain requires.

Nuts and seeds – These aren't just great snacks, they're also bountiful sources of vitamin E and that helps with lessening the amount of cognitive decline as you age. An ounce a day of different varieties such as hazelnuts, walnuts, filberts, Brazil nuts, cashews, almonds, sunflower seeds, peanuts, flax seeds, sesame see as well different nut butters would certainly help. The best bit is that there are a number of different options to choose from too if you're on a diet that restricts certain things.

Whole grains – Oatmeal, whole grain bread as well as brown rice are known to help keep your heart healthy. What you're not often told is that it is also great for your brain. Consider this: Every organ in our body largely depends on proper blood flow in order to function properly. This, of course, includes our brain. Whole grains also contain vitamin E and omega-3 fatty acids which, as you have learned, are great for proper brain function as well. A slice of whole grain bread 2 to 3 times a day or 2 tablespoons of wheat germ a day would provide you with what you need from it.

Chapter 7: Superfoods Recipes With Coconut Oil

In this chapter, we'll help you introduce coconut oil as well as a few other superfoods into your daily diet. For breakfast, snacks, lunch, dinner and even dessert, you'll be able to learn the different ways you can use coconut oil for preparing your meals.

Coconut and Oatmeal Pancakes (Serves 2)

Ingredients:

- ¼ cup coconut flour
- ½ cup coconut milk
- ½ cup oatmeal
- 1 egg
- Some salt
- Coconut Oil for cooking
- Maple syrup for topping

Directions

- Combine your flour, oatmeal, milk, egg and salt in a bowl.
- Using a pan, heat 1 teaspoon of coconut oil before adding ¼ of your coconut flour mixture to it. Cook as preferred.
- Serve warm and top with maple syrup

Hawaiian Rice Medley (Serves 6)

Ingredients:

- 2 cups of organic brown rice
- 4 cups of water
- ¼ cup raw macadamia nuts
- ½ cup fresh mango
- ¼ cup fresh parsley
- ¼ cup fresh cilantro
- 2 tablespoons of pineapple juice concentrate
- ½ teaspoon of salt
- 1/3 cup of toasted coconut flakes

Directions

- A day before serving time (or at least a few hours prior), prepare your rice. To do this, take a large pot and boil water in it before adding your rice. Cook this (don't stir!) for about 40 minutes or until the rice becomes tender. Remove from the heat and stir in your coconut oil. Refrigerate after.
- Before serving, chop up your mangoes, parsley, macadamia nuts and cilantro. Add this to your rice and top with salt and pineapple juice.
- Serve the dish at room temperature.

Kale Chips (Serves 2)

Ingredients:

- 6 cups of kale chips, torn into 1 inch pieces. (Add more as preferred)
- 2 tablespoons of virgin coconut oil
- ¼ teaspoon of salt

Make:

- Start by preheating your oven to 325F
- Rinse your kale and make sure it dries thoroughly. Set aside.
- Pour some of the coconut oil over the kale. Make sure the oil is slightly warm.
- Toss and make sure everything is coated evenly.
- Spread it on a baking sheet, add some salt then bake for at least 20 minutes.

Almond Butter Fudge (Fills and 8x8 pan)

Ingredients:

- 2 cups of creamy almond butter
- ½ cup of coconut oil
- 3 tablespoons of raw honey
- 1 teaspoon salt

Directions

- Mix all of your ingredients together until it becomes smooth and creamy.
- Pour this into a baking dish lined with wax paper. Smooth it out with a spatula before freezing it.

- But into squares and serve immediately.

Green Smoothie With Coconut Oil (Serves 1)

Ingredients:

- A handful of spinach leaves
- 1 tablespoon of ground golden flax seeds
- 1 scoop of mint antioxidant omega 3 greens
- 1 ½ of milk
- 1 scoop of chocolate goat milk protein
- 1 frozen banana, sliced
- 1 teaspoon of virgin coconut oil

Directions

Combine all of your ingredients together in a blender and mix until smooth.

Penne Pasta Salad (Serves 2)

Ingredients:

- 4 tablespoons of coconut oil
- 1 lb of penne pasta, cooked
- ½ cup of red onion, diced
- 2 to 3 cloves garlic, minced
- ¼ cup of red, green and yellow pepper, diced
- ½ a cup of fresh basil
- ¼ cup chopped sun dried tomatoes in olive oil

- Parmesan cheese
- Salt and pepper for seasoning

Directions

- Start by preparing and cooking your pasta then set it aside.
- Heat your coconut oil in a pan, and then add your onion and garlic.
- Add fresh basil and pepper. Cook until it becomes tender.
- Remove these from the heat and add to your pasta.
- Stirring everything well, add the tomatoes and then season with salt and pepper.
- Top with some parmesan cheese.

Thai Chicken Coconut Soup (Serves 4)

Ingredients:

- 8 ounce of mushrooms
- 2 green onions
- 15 oz baby corn, drained
- 1 pound chicken
- 14 ounces of bamboo shoots, drained
- 2 tablespoons of coconut oil
- 1 cup of coconut cream concentrate (Add 2 cups of water)
- 2 chicken bouillon cubes
- 1 teaspoon curry powder
- ½ tablespoon honey
- 2 teaspoon lemon juice
- Salt for seasoning

Directions

- Chop your mushrooms, onions and bamboo shoots into small pieces. Do the same with your chicken before frying it with the coconut oil.
- Add your remaining ingredients and allow it to boil.
- Let it simmer for 15 minutes.

Chapter 8: Coconut Oil Natural Remedies

Besides food, coconut oil is also often used to treat different ailments that a person may experience. In this chapter, we'll provide you with information as well as instructions on how to do just that.

Fungal Treatment

Coconut oil has anti-fungal properties. It can be used topically for: athletes' foot, yeast infections, which include candida. Since it's all natural, you can use it for both adults as well as newborns. It is gentle but effective. All you need to do is take a small amount and apply it directly to the problem area. Do make sure that you clean the spot first to prevent further infection. Do this every day and you'll soon see significant improvement.

Pain Relief

When it comes to alleviating pain, coconut oil works well too. It anti-inflammatory properties are great for getting relief from the symptoms of arthritis. For many people who have this problem, having a natural remedy for their pain is certainly a godsend. After all, a lot of them are not too keen on having to take medication each time their arthritis flares up. With coconut oil, they are able to get relief for their pain and at the same time, boost their overall health. The same applies to other conditions that affect the joints and the bones. A couple of tablespoons a day would be more than enough to help with it.

Allergy Relief

There are a number of different ways through which a person can ease allergic reactions naturally. Coconut oil is among the best remedies for these whether you suffer from the allergies seasonally or chronically. It can even help you deal with any food allergies that you have. However, it should also be noted that there are people who are allergic towards coconut oil itself so if you've never had it before, a quick test should help you determine whether you have it or not. As for treating your allergies with it, adding it to a warm drink such as tea would be the best way of ingesting it.

These are just three of the most common uses for coconut oil as a natural remedy. There are plenty more which you'll eventually discover for yourself as you continue using it.

Chapter 9: Coconut Oil Beauty Recipes

Eager to get started with using coconut oil as a part of your beauty regimen? Here are a few recipes that would help you get started. The ingredients we've chosen for all of these are all-natural and organic so you need not worry about experiencing ill side effects. However, do be wary if you have allergies to some of them.

Homemade Vanilla Nourishing Lip Balm/Salve

Ingredients:

Beeswax, coconut oil and vanilla extract

Directions:

- Melt your beeswax and coconut oil over a double boiler. Put more beeswax than coconut oil to make sure your balm is firm.
- Remove from the heat and allow to cool for a bit before adding your vanilla extract.
- Transfer this to an old lip balm tube or tin. Refrigerate.

Coconut Oil Healing Face Mask

Ingredients:

Honey and coconut oil

Directions:

- Mix the two in equal amounts. Just enough to cover your face.
- Apply evenly and massage into your skin for a few minutes.
- Rinse with warm water and your favorite facial cleanser.

Body Moisturizing Whipped Lotion

Ingredients:

Coconut oil, jojoba oil and your favorite essential oil

Directions:

- Melt and mix your two oils together in equal amounts. Allow to cool a bit, and then add your favorite essential oil.
- Set aside and allow it to turn opaque. Bring out your mixer and whip until it takes on the appearance of whipped cream.
- Store in a sanitized container and keep away from heat.

Exfoliating Body Scrub

Ingredients:

Coconut oil and brown sugar

Directions:

- Add a tablespoon of brown sugar to 3 tablespoons of coconut oil. You can make more as needed.
- Apply liberally to your problem spots and work it in before rinsing off with warm water.

Deep Conditioner for Healthier and Smoother Hair

Ingredients:

3 to 5 tablespoons of coconut oil

Directions:

- If you're working with a solid version of the oil, melt over warm heat and allow to cool but not to harden.
- Work this into your hair, starting with the tips before making your way to your scalp.
- Leave on for half an hour before rinsing it off.

These are just a few simple recipes that you can try at home when it comes to using coconut oil for your skin and hair. With constant use, you're sure to find more uses for it. Since it's all natural and contains no harsh chemicals, you can use it on younger children as well as babies without any worry.

Chapter 10: Choosing The Right Coconut Oil

Not sure about which variety of coconut oil to choose for your needs? Well, don't fret! In this chapter, we'll provide you with the information you need to know when it comes to differentiating one type from the other.

Unrefined

This is considered by many to be the best and healthiest variety. Unrefined refers to "virgin" coconut oil which hasn't undergone any process and isn't altered chemically. There are varieties that have been refined, bleached and deodorized which can actually remove or even reverse some of the health benefits.

Do keep in mind that processed coconut oil is not meant for consumption and is often solely relegated to industrial use. Always go for virgin or extra virgin coconut oil when buying some.

Non-Hydrogenated

Keep away from this one as well! It becomes quite unstable when placed at high temperatures and has lost its essential fatty acid components In fact, instead of the good fat, you'll find trans fats instead. These are the top culprits for obesity as well as heart disease.

Cold Pressed

How can you make sure that the oil you're purchasing still retains its health benefits? Well, go for cold pressed. This process makes sure that no heat is unnecessarily added to the oil thus making sure that its benefits remain uncompromised. The downside is that it tends to be more expensive than your average coconut oil but it certainly is worth it.

Conclusion

Thank you again for purchasing this book *Coconut Oil: Ultimate Coconut Oil Guide! - Coconut Oil Recipes for Organic Skin Care and Natural Beauty, Clean Eating for Weight Loss, Shining Hair, Better Brain Function and Overall Health!*

I am extremely excited to pass this information along to you, and I am so happy that you now have read and can hopefully implement these strategies going forward.

I hope this book was able to help you understand what makes coconut oil special when it comes to benefitting not your just your health but your physical appearance. We also hope that through the recipes provided, you'll be enticed to try it out for yourself thus allowing you to experience it first-hand.

The next step is to get started using this information and to hopefully lead a healthier, better and more efficient life! All thanks to the changes that coconut oil will help bring about. Please don't be someone who just reads this information and doesn't apply it, the strategies in this book will only benefit you if you use them!

If you know of anyone else that could benefit from the information presented here please inform them of this book.

Finally, if you enjoyed this book and feel it has added value to your life in any way, please take the time to share your thoughts and post a review on Amazon. It'd be greatly appreciated!

Thank you and good luck!

Preview Of:

Ultimate Mindful Eating Guide!

<u>Mindful Eating</u>

Stop Overeating And Binge Eating For Good And Lose Weight With Mindfulness, Self Discipline, Meditation, And Willpower Strategies!

Introduction

I want to thank you and congratulate you for purchasing the book, *"Mindful Eating: Ultimate Mindful Eating Guide! - Stop Overeating And Binge Eating For Good And Lose Weight With Mindfulness, Self Discipline, Meditation, And Willpower Strategies!"*

This Mindfulness Eating book contains proven steps and strategies on how to avoid overeating and binge eating for good. It is easy to fall into the trap of mindless eating especially given the world's culture today, but it does not mean that overeating should be a normal part of life.

Overeating and binge eating can lead to serious health problems and issues, and it is time that people take an active stance against such issues. Lead a healthy and well-balanced life by following simple steps and strategies that will keep you off your cravings and away from binge eating.

Thanks again for purchasing this book, I hope you enjoy it!

Chapter 1: What Does Mindful Eating Mean? What Does Binge Eating Mean?

Eating is a natural way of life. People, along with all the other animals and living things in the world need to eat or consume foods in order to grow and survive. However, there is more to eating than simply shoving up food into our mouths.

Mindful Eating

In the world today where food seems to be everywhere, the act of eating becomes what is known as a mindless deed. There is hardly any thought that goes along with the action and many people seem to just eat whatever food is right before them. In some cases, people are not even aware of the foods that they consume or would simply forget about them mere minutes after they have eaten. These facts tell us that the act of mindless eating is so rampant that it oftentimes leads to guilt and weight and health related problems. If there is such a thing as mindless eating, what is mindful eating then?

To some, mindful eating is the act of being fully aware of and in control of what they eat. This means that they pay every attention to the foods they eat and are therefore able to notice and enjoy every bite they take. It also means being aware of the foods' effects on the body, and therefore having the intention of taking care of oneself. After all, no one would mindfully eat something if there is a known negative effect on the self. To this respect, mindful eating builds a peaceful relationship with the body where the body's needs and sometimes even the wants, are satisfied. It becomes an act of wisdom and of full consciousness as it chooses what is natural and healthy.

Binge Eating

On the other end of the spectrum is what is known as binge eating. This is the earlier form of eating that was discussed as being mindless, and even sometimes taken to an extreme level. Binge eating is defined as disordered eating wherein the act is uncontrollable. This leads to eating enormous amounts of food even after the individual has had the feeling of a full stomach.

Most people who suffer from binge eating try to hide it from friends and family, leading them to isolate themselves in many instances.

In extreme cases, binge eating is a serious disorder where one consumes unusually excessive amounts of food. Even those who are not diagnosed with the disorder can experience occasional bouts of binge eating where they find themselves unable to restrain themselves from eating. In some books, the definition of binge eating is excessive and uncontrollable eating that is followed by feelings of guilt and shame. This compulsive eating disorder also leads to many weight and health problems including but not limited to obesity and excessive weight gain. Women have been found to make up 60% of those with binge eating symptoms and one in every five women have reported to experiencing symptoms of binge eating.

Thanks for Previewing My Exciting Book Entitled:

"Mindful Eating: Ultimate Mindful Eating Guide! Stop Overeating And Binge Eating For Good And Lose Weight With Mindfulness, Self Discipline, Meditation, And Willpower Strategies!"

To purchase this book, simply go to the Amazon Kindle store and simply search:

"MINDFUL EATING"

Then just scroll down until you see my book. You will know it is mine because you will see my name "Sarah Brooks" underneath the title.

Alternatively, you can visit my author page on Amazon to see this book and other work I have done. Thanks so much, and please don't forget your free bonuses

DON'T LEAVE YET! - CHECK OUT YOUR FREE BONUSES BELOW!

Free Bonus Offer: Get Free Access To The www.LuxyLifeNaturals.com VIP Newsletter!

Once you enter your email address you will immediately get free access to this awesome newsletter!

But wait, right now if you join now for free you will also get free access to the "Anti-Aging Made Easy" free EBook!

To claim both your FREE VIP NEWSLETTER MEMBERSHIP and your FREE BONUS Ebook on ANTI-AGING MADE EASY!

Just Go To:

www.LuxyLifeNaturals.com

www.ingramcontent.com/pod-product-compliance
Lightning Source LLC
Chambersburg PA
CBHW070933290526
45795CB00003B/1007